I0421992

Ultimate Superfoods Health And Diet Detox Guide!

<u>Superfoods</u>

Increase Metabolism, Natural Beauty And Health With 50 Powerful Remedies And Recipes For Anti-Aging, Fat Loss, And More!

Sarah Brooks

Copyright © 2014 Sarah Brooks

STOP!!! Before you read any further....Would you like to know the secrets of Anti-Aging?

If your answer is yes, then you are not alone. Thousands of people are looking for the secret to reducing wrinkles, looking younger, and maintaining a youthful appearance.

If you have been searching for these answers without much luck, you are in the right place!

Not only will you gain incredible insight in this book, but because I want to make sure to give you as much value as possible, right now for a limited time you can get full **100% FREE access to a VIP bonus eBook** entitled **Anti-Aging Made Easy!**

Just Go Here For Free Instant Access:

www.LuxyLifeNaturals.com

Legal Notice

All rights reserved. Without limiting the rights under the copyright reserved above, no part of this publication may be reproduced, stored in or introduced into a retrieval system, or transmitted, in any form, or by any means (electronic, mechanical, photocopying, recording, or otherwise) without the prior written permission of the copyright owner and publisher of this book. This book is copyright protected. This is for your personal use only. You cannot amend, distribute, sell, use, quote or paraphrase any part or the content within this eBook without the consent of the author or copyright owner. Legal action will be pursued if this is breached.

Disclaimer Notice

Please note the information contained within this document is for educational and entertainment purposes only. Considerable energy and every attempt has been made to provide the most up to date, accurate, relative, reliable, and complete information, but the reader is strongly encouraged to seek professional advice prior to using any of this information contained in this book. The reader understands they are reading and using this information contained herein at their own risk, and in no way will the author, publisher, or any affiliates be held responsible for any damages whatsoever. No warranties of any kind are expressed or implied. Readers acknowledge that the author is not engaging in the rendering of legal, financial, medical, or any other professional advice. By reading this document, the reader agrees that under no circumstances is the author, publisher, or anyone else affiliated with the production, distribution, sale, or any other element of this book responsible for any losses, direct or indirect, which are incurred as a result of the use of information contained within this document, including, but not limited to, errors, omissions, or inaccuracies. Because of the rate with which conditions change, the author and publisher reserve the right to alter and update the information contained herein on the new conditions whenever they see applicable.

Table Of Contents

Introduction

I want to thank you and congratulate you for purchasing the book, *Superfoods: Ultimate Superfoods Health And Diet Detox Guide! - Increase Metabolism, Natural Beauty And Health With 50 Powerful Natural Remedies And Recipes For Anti-Aging, Fat Loss, And More!.*

This book contains proven steps and strategies on how to use superfoods to achieve the best health. Superfoods have a tons of benefits in the body. Metabolism is increased and the body is detoxified, which improves organ functioning. They also can greatly help with weight loss and reduce inflammation, among many other amazing benefits!

In this book you will learn much more about these superfoods, and also how you can create healthy meals out of these foods!

Thanks again for purchasing this book, I hope you enjoy it!

Chapter 1: What Are Superfoods And How Can They Help You?

Superfoods are foods that have been informally named for their multiple and wide ranging health benefits. These are foods that are packed with nutrients that have very potent effects on the body.

These foods are mostly plant-based. However, some fish and dairy are also included in this food group. Superfoods are so-named because they are nutritionally dense. That is, there have high levels of vitamins and minerals that support health. In addition to these, they are also packed with special compounds. They have provide rich supplies of antioxidants that rid the body of free radicals and toxins, detoxify the liver and other organs, and protects tissues from damage. They also have compounds that have anticancer properties.

Superfoods are also rich in trace elements that support several bodily functions. They accelerate certain enzyme actions to boost health.

These foods also have an abundance of compounds that have potent anti-cancer properties. They protect the body from damage that can trigger the development of cancer. They also strengthen the immune system to fight off cancer-causing compounds and infections.

Other benefits from superfoods include strengthening the tissues. They also improve blood flow to the tissues. Blood brings oxygen and nutrients to the cells. t also takes cell debris and wastes out of the tissues and to the excretory organs. Good blood flow means good efficient exchange of nutrients and wastes. This way, the body gets to function more efficiently.

Superfoods also strengthen the digestive system. This way, food is better digested, absorbed ad delivered to the different tissues.

There are also a lot more benefits from the many compounds in the different superfoods. Just take care to consume in moderation. Some superfoods include fruits that have sugar and fats in them.

Overconsumption can cause imbalance, despite the many health benefits.

Chapter 2: 20 Superfoods For A Diet Detox And Health Rejuvenation

Detoxifying the body helps to remove accumulated toxins and free radicals. It also helps to clear the body of sludge that slows down its functions.

Lemon

Lemon is also one of the best superfoods for detoxifying the liver. It contains large amounts of vitamin C that the body converts into glutathione, which the Phase 2 of liver detoxification needs.

Cabbage

Cabbage has several compounds that have anti-cancer and antioxidant properties. These compounds aid the liver in breaking down substances in the body for excretion, like excess hormones. Cabbage can neutralize toxic compounds from exposure to cigarette smoke. They also stimulate the liver to release more enzymes used for detox.

Garlic

Garlic has antimicrobial properties that helps cleanse the body from viruses, parasites and bacteria. It has an abundance of antioxidant and anticancer compounds that help detoxify the body.

Almonds

Almonds are superfoods that are rich in fiber, magnesium, proteins and calcium. These compounds help to rid the digestive system of toxins. They also help stabilize the levels of blood sugar.

Beetroot

Beets are abundant in minerals and phytochemicals that work together to fight infection, purify the blood and cleanse the liver. It also helps to stabilize the acid-base balance of the blood, which supports detoxification.

Avocado

Avocados are contains the compound glutathione that plays an important role in liver detoxification process.

Blueberries

These superfruits are rich in proanthocyanidins, which have potent detoxifying effects.

Cranberries

These berries help detoxify and cleanse the body, by helping to flush out infective microorganisms from the urinary tract.

Kale

The antioxidants help get rid of the toxins in the body. It has an active compound that neutralizes harmful compounds from cigarette smoke. It also has a compound that helps in stimulating the liver to produce and release detoxifying enzymes.

Dandelion

This "weed" has long been used to improve liver health.

Ginger

More popularly taken as tea and is long believed to help the liver function better

Grapefruit

Has an abundance of antioxidants that help in detoxifying the body. It floods the body with an abundance of good nutrients that push the bad ones from the tissues

Lemongrass

Helps in cleansing several organs at the same time, such as the liver and kidneys

Olive oil

Has potent purging effects that stimulates the liver and the gall bladder to remove gall bladder stones

Seaweed

Receives little attention but the nori in sushi is packed with antioxidants that detoxify the body

Turmeric

A spice often taken as tea to detoxify

Wheatgrass

Potent detoxifier as to boost liver functioning

Artichokes

Helps in the liver function, which accelerates the excretion of toxins

Asparagus

Antioxidant and other phytochemicals help in detoxifying the body

Chapter 3: 20 Superfoods For Increasing Metabolism And Ramping Up Weight Loss

Superfoods also boost the metabolism. By increasing the rate of metabolism, weight can be effectively controlled.

Apple cider vinegar

The compounds suppress the appetite.

Greek yogurt

This is a good substitute to most dairy needs and requirements. It is also a healthier and more filling superfood. It is packed with protein and with much less sugar.

Olive oil

It is a healthy alternative to salad dressings. This healthy fat can coat the cells and help to metabolize fats and keep the weight off.

Turkey breast

Good protein source and helps to rev up the metabolism to keep weight off.

Quinoa

Helps in regulating the blood sugar levels, which helps in regulating weight gain

Leafy greens

The phytochemicals and antioxidants help speed up metabolism and boost energy. They are also rich in fiber than helps inn curbing appetite and feel full longer

Oat

They are rich in fiber that helps feel full longer. They also help improve the body's lipid profile that helps with weight loss.

Pineapple

Contains phytochemicals that increases the rate of metabolism and keeps the cardiovascular system healthy.

Cayenne pepper

Capsaicin stimulates higher metabolic rates

Other fruits that boost metabolism from its many vitamins and minerals, not to mention its high fiber content:

- Banana
- Kiwi
- Orange
- Lemon
- Lime
- Apple
- Pear
- Blueberries

Herbs that can boost metabolism and promote weight loss

- Red bell pepper
- Rosemary
- Cinnamon
- Turmeric
- Mint

.

Chapter 4: 20 Superfoods To Eat For Natural Beauty And A Youthful Complexion

Beauty can be achieved naturally with superfoods, which are packed with vitamins, omega-3 fatty acids, minerals and antioxidants. They get rid of toxins, support healthy cells and keep the body functioning at its best.

Spinach

Spinach is a leafy green that is rich in lutein, vitamins (B, C and E), antioxidants, omega-3 fats and minerals (magnesium, calcium, potassium, iron). This can be used in place of lettuce for healthier benefits.

Wild Salmon

Salmon is rich in antioxidants and omega-3 fats. It keeps the skin well moisturized and supple. It is also rich in selenium, which has protective properties that shield the skin from sun damage. Vitamin D is also present in wild salmon, which helps keep strong bones and teeth.

Low-fat Dairy Products

These foods are rich in vitamin A. This is a key component that helps the skin cells in proper maturation and development. Low fat dairy product includes plain yogurt and Greek yogurt.

Flaxseed

This superfood can delay the appearance of wrinkles. It contains large amounts of the good kind of fats, omega-3 fatty acids. These beneficial fats strengthen the cell membranes. By this, the cells have a reinforcement, which makes it more difficult for harmful substances to pass through the cell membrane. Also, it keeps moisture in. These actions when targeted to the skin cells means it becomes suppler, softer, better texture and clearer. When more cells hold water longer, the skin looks younger and plumper.

Green tea

This kind of tea contains a good amount of polyphenols. It prevents skin damage. In addition, it also has potent antioxidant and anti-inflammatory.

Tuna

This is the superfood for sagging skin. Tuna has an abundance of nutrients, particularly selenium. It prevents skin cellular damage that may come from exposure to the sun, toxins, elements and other harmful substances. Selenium also promotes the production of the protein elastin. This protein promotes flexibility, smoothness and tightness of the skin.

Avocado

Avocado improves the skin's elasticity because of its abundance of monounsaturated fats. The fats reinforce the cell membranes of skin cells, which make them stronger and better at resisting damage and wrinkling.

Tomatoes

Lycopene in tomatoes are released during the cooking process. This compound aids in defending the skin cells against damage from sun exposure. It also helps to prevent premature aging and wrinkles. It can also neutralize the harmful effects of UV radiation.

Sweet Potatoes

Sweet potatoes contain an excellent amount of vitamin C. This vitamin plays an important role in collagen development. Collagen is an important protein that contributes to skin elasticity. More vitamin C means more collagen production. The skin becomes more youthful looking and fuller. It also prevents the premature appearance of wrinkles.

Berries

Berries help protect the skin from sun damage. They are rich in flavones, which helps keep the skin look healthier and younger.

Almonds

Almonds are rich in vitamin E, one of the many compounds that act as natural sun blocks. Antioxidant vitamins, they are called, are effective in blocking the UV radiations and protecting the skin cells from sun damage that includes premature aging and wrinkles.

Foods rich in selenium

Other superfoods that you should be eating to help the skin achieve a youthful complexion are those that are high in selenium. This mineral promotes faster cell turnover to replace old and damaged skin cells. They also help in keeping the cells healthier. Foods include the following:

- whole-grain cereals
- whole-wheat muffins and breads
- turkey

- brazil nuts
- tuna

Chapter 5: 15 Superfoods To Apply To Your Skin For Natural Beauty And Slowing Down The Aging Process

Skin health can be made better with superfoods. It is more of a cumulative effect from the many actions of superfoods. The antioxidants detoxify the blood and promote better blood flow. This results in better skin nourishment. Good blood flow means better skin nourishment. The skin cells will develop faster and better, replacing old and aged cells better. The skin would look glowing and younger.

Tomatoes

This superfood contains the potent compound lycopene. It has potent antioxidant properties with an anti-aging effect to the skin. Lycopene is better absorbed when the tomatoes are cooked.

Rosemary

This herb has protective properties that keep the skin from premature aging.

Red bell pepper

This provides a good amount of vitamin C, which prevent premature skin aging. Eating more red bell peppers reduces the appearance of skin dryness, thinning and wrinkles.

Pineapple

Phytochemicals in pineapple protects against free radical damage that can cause premature aging. It is also rich in vitamin C that aids in skin health. It also contains bromelain, a compound that helps the skin heal faster for younger looking and sin and for better complexion.

Butternut squash

Beta carotene in butternut squash protects the skin cells from UV damage, which causes wrinkles and age spots.

Walnuts

Compounds in walnuts help to soothe dry and irritated skin. It is also rich in omega-3 fats that helps reduce redness in the skin and keep moisture in.

Dark berries like cherries and blackberries

These are high in vitamin C and antioxidants, which protects the skin cells from damage caused by free radicals.

Coconut water

Coconut water helps hydrate the skin. It also helps to plump the skin cells to improve complexion and for younger-looking skin. Potassium in coconut water can also help cleanse the skin.

Acerola cherry juice

Hydrate the skin by drinking lots f fluids, including this juice. It is rich in vitamin A and vitamin that are important for smooth and clear skin complexion. It is also high in vitamin C that reduces fine lines and wrinkles. It also helps plump the skin.

Avocados

Is an amazing skin food because of the monounsaturated fats and vitamins (A, D and E) that nourish the skin

Radishes

Rich in vitamin, silicon and sulfur that boosts collagen production in the skin. They also help make the skin glow.

Watercress

The compounds in watercress serve as internal skin cleanser and antiseptic.

Pumpkin seeds

It is high in zinc. This mineral effectively promotes skin health. It controls oil production and regulates hormones that contribute to acne.

Green tea

Rich in antioxidants that protects against free radical damage. It also reduces fine lines and wrinkles. It also contains polyphenols that help revive old and dying skin cells.

Chapter 6: 20 Superfoods For Brain Health And Focus

The brain also benefits from the compounds in superfoods. These foods can increase and improve blood flow to the brain. Better blood flow gives better nourishment to the brain cells, which function better. Better concentration and focus, better judgment, improved learning and memory skills are just some of the benefits.

Whole Grains

These foods are abundant in fiber, minerals, phytonutrients and vitamins. They promote good blood flow to the organs, including the brain. Brown rice is a good choice.

Tea

Green tea is high in EGCG, a polyphenol that prevents the degradation of neurotransmitters in the brain. This means better and higher brain activity.

White tea is made from young tea leaves and underwent less processing. This means it retains more of its natural catechin. This potent antioxidant reverses and prevents any abnormality in cellular growth.

Blueberries

The antioxidant compounds prevent oxidative stress in the brain. In turn, it provides some degree of protection against brain degenerative disorders such as Alzheimer's disease. It can also improve learning and memory.

Citrus

Citrus fruits like lemons, grapefruit and oranges are rich in Vitamin C. It plays a role in the production of neurotransmitters that help the rain function better.

Dark chocolate

Dark chocolate, at least 70% cacao, contains flavonoid antioxidants. These substances improve blood flow to the brain.

Flaxseed and its oil

These are rich in essential fatty acids that are critical in maintaining brain health.

Milk

It is abundant in B vitamins that help and support the memory function.

Spinach

This vegetable has high levels of magnesium, which plays an important role in the circuitry of the brain.

Squash

This vegetable is rich in B12 and folic acid that prevents the cells from shrinking.

Potato

High levels of vitamin B6 support the body's serotonin levels and stabilize patterns of sleep.

Broccoli

The compound sulforaphane in broccoli has a protective function on the blood-brain capillaries.

Wheat germ

This superfood helps prevent strokes because if the high amounts of vitamin B-complex.

Mango, Pomegranate

Supports the mood through its abundance of amino acids

Honey

Has high levels of fructose that provide fuel to brain cells

Beans and legumes

Rich in essential fatty acids and folate that supports brain function

Coconut oil

Contains medium chain triglycerides that the body readily uses. This way, glucose becomes more available for the brain cells to use.

Nuts

They are rich in essential fats like omega-3 and omega-6, vitamin E and vitamin B6 that protects the brain from free radical damage. It also improves brain power.

Rosemary

This herb improves cognitive and memory function just by its scent. As food, it can improve the blood flow towards the brain. It also improves mood.

Sunflower seeds

Contains tryptophan, a compound that the brain converts into the neurotransmitter serotonin. This neurotransmitter boosts mood and helps in controlling depression.

Quinoa

Serves as a healthy glucose source that fuels the brain

Chapter 7: Superfoods Recipes To Decrease Inflammation And Heal Your Body

Inflammation is damaging to the body. It is important to decrease inflammation so that the body can concentrate on healing itself. Without inflammation, the body can repair and rejuvenate tissues and organs to improve functioning.

Baby Cabbage and Almonds Salad With Garlic and Malt Mayo Dressing

Ingredients (makes 4 servings):

- 2 heads of baby cabbages, sliced very thinly (julienned)
- 8 pieces of baby carrots, peeled then shaved
- ½ cup almonds, roughly chopped
- A pinch of red chilli (dried), for toppings

For the mayonnaise:

- 2 teaspoon Dijon mustard
- 1 medium sized free-range egg
- 2 cloves of garlic, chopped finely
- 1 tablespoon of malt vinegar
- ½ cup of canola oil
- Sea salt, to taste
- Black pepper, freshly ground, to taste

Preparation:

- Toss the cabbage, carrots and dates together in a large mixing bowl.

- Place all the mayonnaise ingredients, except the oil, in a blender. Blend until all ingredients are well combined. While still blending, slowly pour the oil into the mixture. Continue blending until the oil is fully incorporated into the mixture.

- Add the mayonnaise to the vegetables and mix until everything is lightly coated.

- Sprinkle dried chili and serve.

Hot Beetroot, Citrus and Coriander Mixed Drink

Ingredients (makes 4 to 6 servings):

- 500 grams punnet of beetroot, cooked

- Extracted juice of 3 medium-sized lemon

- 1 cup of vegetable stock

- 1 tablespoon of honey

- Fresh coriander leaves, about a handful

- Sea salt

- Pepper, freshly ground

Preparation:

- Chop the beetroot roughly.

- Mix all the ingredients together in a blender. Process until it achieves a smooth consistency.

- Place the pot over medium fire and heat through.

- Season with salt and pepper to taste.

- Add more stock as necessary until the consistency is good for sipping.

Creamy Citrusy Avocado Coleslaw

Ingredients (makes 2 servings):

- 2 heads of baby cabbage, sliced into shreds

- 2 medium sized baby carrots, peel and shred

- 1 piece large and ripe avocado

- 1 clove of garlic, crushed

- ¾ cup of crème fraiche

- Sea salt and black pepper, to taste

Preparation:

- Toss all the ingredients in a large mixing bowl, except the avocado.

- Slice the avocado in thin strips.

- Once everything is evenly mixed, gently fold in the avocado. Be careful not to mash the fruit.

- Serve. Squeeze half a lemon, if desired.

Pear with Ricotta and Cinnamon

Ingredients (makes 1 serving):

- 1 small-sized pear, cored and halved
- ¼ cup ricotta cheese, part skim
- ¼ teaspoon of ground cinnamon

Preparation:

- Preheat a toaster or a broiler.
- Arrange the pear on a shallow baking pan.
- Broil the pear until tender, for about 10-12 minutes.
- In a small bowl, mix the cheese and cinnamon.
- When the pear is ready, top the halves with the cheese mixture.

Amaranth Porridge

Ingredients (makes 2 servings):

- 2/3 cup whole grain amaranth
- 2 cups filtered water
- 1 tablespoon raw honey
- ¼ cup pumpkin seeds or hemp

- 1 teaspoon cinnamon

- ½ cup dried cranberries or blueberries

- 1 medium-sized pear

Preparation:

- Place the amaranth and water in a pot with a tight lid.

- Bring to a boil. Then lower the heat.

- Stir frequently to prevent the porridge from sticking.

- Cook until the liquids are absorbed.

- Remove from heat and add all the rest of the ingredients.

Crispy Kale Chips

Ingredients (makes 8 servings):

- 2 large bunches of kale leaves

- 1 cup sweet potatoes, grated

- 1 cup fresh cashews

- 2 tablespoon nutritional yeast

- Juice of 1 lemon

- 1 tablespoon raw honey

- 2 tablespoon filtered water

- ½ teaspoon salt

Preparation:

- Remove the stems from the kale leaves and place them in a large mixing bowl.

- Place all the remaining ingredients in a blender. Process until the mixture becomes smooth.

- Pour the mixture over the kale leaves. Mix thoroughly to coat the leaves evenly.

- Arrange the coated kale leaves in a single layer on a baking sheet.

- Dehydrate the leaves in the oven set at 150 degrees. This takes about 2 hours.

- Turn the leaves while baking to ensure the leaves dry evenly.

- Remove the leaves and cool. Store in airtight container. Eat as snack or as side dish.

Beet Salad

Ingredients (makes 4 servings):

- 1 large beet, grated coarsely

- 1 large apple, cored and diced

- 1 large carrot, grated coarsely

- 2 tablespoon almonds, chopped

- 2 tablespoon lemon juice

- 2 tablespoon flax or pumpkin seed oil

- 4 cup mixed greens

Preparation:

- Toss everything in large bowl, except the mixed greens.

- Arrange the mixed greens on a plate. Spoon the apple mixture over the greens and serve.

Noodle-less Pad Thai

Ingredients (makes 4 servings):

- 1 medium sized zucchini

- 1 large carrot

- 1 piece green onion, chopped

- ½ cup of cauliflower florets

- ½ cup purple cabbage, shredded

- ½ cup radish or mung bean sprouts

Sauce:

- 2 tablespoon tahini

- 1 tablespoon lime or lemon juice

- 2 tablespoon almond butter

- 1 tablespoon raw honey

- 2 tablespoon wheat-free tamari

- ½ teaspoon grated ginger root

- ¼ teaspoon minced garlic

Preparation:

- Create the "noodles" from carrots and zucchini. Pass a peeler over these vegetables or use a mandolin.

- Place the "noodles" in a large bowl.

- Add the other vegetables: cabbage, cauliflower, radish (or mung bean sprouts) and green onion.

- In a separate bowl, mix all the ingredients for the sauce.

- Pour the sauce of the vegetables and toss gently.

- Serve immediately but for best flavors, serve the next day to allow the flavors time to blend and settle.

Beef Tenderloin with Spice Rub

Ingredients (makes 4 servings):

- 4 pieces of 6-ounce beef tenderloin filets

- 2 sprigs of fresh rosemary

- 2 tablespoon garlic, minced

- 2 teaspoon cumin seeds (lightly dry-toasted and ground)

- 2 teaspoon coriander seeds (lightly dry-toasted and ground)

- 1 teaspoon cinnamon

- ½ teaspoon allspice

- 1 teaspoon minced fresh ginger root

- ½ teaspoon salt

Preparation:

- In a small bowl, mix garlic, spices, rosemary, salt and ginger. Set aside.

- Arrange the meat fillet in a baking dish. Coat both side of the eat with the spice mixture.

- Broil the meat 6 inches from the heat. Cook about 4-6 minutes in each side, according to preferred doneness.

- Remove when done. Rest the meat before serving.

Kale salad

Ingredients (makes 4 servings):

- 6 cups chopped kale leaves

- ½ of a lemon

- Pinch of basil, dried

- Pinch of salt

- 1 tablespoon of extra-virgin olive oil

- 2 tablespoon minced red onion

- 2 tablespoon chopped green onion

- 1 small cucumber, sliced thinly

- 1 clove garlic, minced

- ¼ cup kalamata olives, chopped

Preparation:

- Wash kale thoroughly then cut them into strips.

- Steam the kale leaves lightly for about 5-7 minutes. Place in a large bowl.

- Add lemon, salt, oil and basil. Toss lightly to mix.

- Add all the remaining ingredients and mix thoroughly.

- Serve.

Baked Cinnamon Apples

Ingredients (makes 4 servings):

- 4 medium sized apples

- ½ cup mixed seeds and/or nuts

- 2 dates, pitted then chopped

- ¼ cup dried cranberries

- 1 teaspoon fresh ginger root, grated

- ½ teaspoon nutmeg

- 1 teaspoon cinnamon

- ¼ teaspoon ground cloves

- 1 cup apple juice (or apple cider)

- ¼ cup honey

Preparation:

- Preheat the oven to 325 degrees Fahrenheit.

- Mix dates, cranberries, nuts (or seeds), spices and ginger in a medium-sized bowl.

- Core the apples but be careful not to but through the bottom.

- Stuff the apples with the nut (or seed) mixture.

- Drizzle with honey.

- Place the apples in a baking dish.

- Pour the juice (or cider) around the fruit to prevent drying during the baking process.

- Bake the apples for 30-35 minutes until the apples are soft.

- Serve the apples warm.

Key Lime Pie

Ingredients (makes 8 servings):

<u>For the crust</u>

- 1 cup coconut (unsweetened), shredded

- 1 cup walnuts

- ¼ teaspoon salt

- ½ cup dates, pitted

<u>For the filling</u>

- 3 pieces avocados

- 3 tablespoon lime juice

- 1 teaspoon lime zest

- ½ cup raw honey

- Pinch salt

- lime or kiwi, as desired

Preparation:

- Place the coconut, salt and walnuts in a food processor. Process until everything is coarsely ground.

- Add the dates to the food processor. Continue processing until the mixture resembles breadcrumbs.

- Press the crust mixture into the bottom of a pie plate.

- Freeze the crust for 15 minutes.

- In the meantime, prepare the filling.

- Place all the filling ingredients in the food processor. Blend until the consistency is smooth.

- Take the crust out and pour the filling in.

- Return to the fridge to set for about 20 minutes.

- When ready to serve, garnish with kiwi or lime slices.

Chapter 8: Superfoods Recipes To Increase Fat Loss

Banana and Nut Pancakes

Ingredients (makes 3 pancakes):

- ½ cup quinoa, cooked

- 2 egg whites

- ½ cup 1% milk

- 1 teaspoon brown sugar

- ¼ teaspoon vanilla

- ½ of a medium-sized banana

  Toppings:

- ½ of a banana

- 2 tablespoon of nonfat, plain Greek yogurt

- 2 tablespoon of walnuts, chopped

- 1 teaspoon maple syrup

Preparation:

- Make the pancake batter. In a large bowl, mix together quinoa, milk, egg whites, vanilla, brown sugar and banana.

- Place a skillet over medium heat. Lightly coat it with vegetable cooking oil spray.

- Carefully pour the batter on the heated skillet. Make 3 pancakes.

- Cook each side until done, flip once. It will take about 3 minutes to cook each side.

- Remove from pan and transfer on a plate.

- Top with ¼ of a banana, walnuts, Greek yogurt and maple syrup.

Weight Loss Smoothie

Ingredients (makes 1 serving):

- 1 cup of almond milk, soy or skim milk

- ½ cup of kale leaves

- 1 small banana

- Almond butter

- A handful of chia seeds

Preparation:

- Place everything in blender and process until smooth and creamy.

Fruit-and-Oat Smoothie

Ingredients (makes 2 servings):

- 1 cup water

- 1 6-ounce of 2% plain Greek yogurt

- ½ cup mango chunks, fresh or frozen

- ½ cup strawberries, fresh or frozen, sliced

- ½ cup ale leaves, chopped

- 1/3 cup rolled oats

Preparation:

- Place all the ingredients in a blender. Puree until everything is well blended, smooth and creamy. Serve.

Grilled Cheese with Kale

Ingredients (makes 1 serving):

- ½ teaspoon minced garlic

- 1 cup kale leaves, sliced thinly

- 1 artichoke heart, chopped

- 2 slices of bread, whole grain variety

- 2 slices 2% cheddar cheese

Preparation:

- Gat a non-stick pan and mist it with cooking spray. Heat it over medium high heat.

- Sauté the garlic, artichoke and kale until the leaves wilt, about 4 minutes.

- Remove from heat and set aside.

- Place the cheese in each slice of bread and top with the kale mixture.

- Place the bread on a skillet and cook over medium heat.

- Cook until the underside of the bread turns gold and the cheese starts to melt.

- Press the bread together to make a sandwich.

- Serve warm.

Baked walnut-crusted Tilapia with Barley, Garlic, Cranberry and Green Beans Salad

Ingredients (makes 2 servings):

- 5 ounces of tilapia
- 2 teaspoons honey Dijon mustard
- 1 tablespoon walnuts, chopped finely
- ¾ cup barley, cooked
- 1 teaspoon apple cider vinegar
- 1 tablespoon dried cranberries
- 1 small green onion, sliced thinly
- 2 teaspoons olive oil
- 1 teaspoon garlic, minced
- 1 cup green beans
- Salt and pepper to taste

Preparation:

- Preheat the oven to 375°F.
- Arrange the fish on a baking sheet lined with foil.
- Spoon the mustard over the fish.
- Sprinkle the walnuts over the fish and press it firmly to the flesh. Bake until done. With a fork, the fish should flake easily.

- Make the salad by mixing the barley, vinegar, cranberries, and onion. Toss them together.

- Sauté the garlic in oil and add the green beans. Cook until the beans are crisp-tender.

- Season to taste with salt and pepper.

- Arrange the fish on a plate and the veggies on the side.

Turkey Chili Fries

Ingredients (makes 2 servings):

- 1 medium potato, cut into ½-inch strips

- 4 ounces 99% fat-free ground turkey

- 1 tablespoon of taco seasoning

- 2 tablespoon of water

- ½ cup green bell pepper, diced

- ¼ cup kidney beans, rinsed and drained

- ¼ cup cheddar cheese, shredded

- ½ cup tomato, diced

- ½ green onion

- 2 tablespoon 2% plain Greek yogurt

Preparation:

- Preheat the oven to 400°F.

- Arrange the potato strips in a single layer on a baking sheet.

- Spray with cooking oil spray, bake in the oven for 30 minutes. Halfway through the baking, flip the potatoes.

- Place a skillet on medium heat.

- Cook the ground turkey. Add the taco seasoning and water. Continue cooking until the turkey is cooked through.

- Add the green bell pepper and beans. Sauté for about 4 minutes.

- To arrange, place the cooked turkey over the potatoes. add the cheese, tomato and onion. Top everything with the Greek yogurt.

Roast Beef with Parmesan and Arugula

Ingredients (makes 2 servings):

- 1 6-inch pita bread, whole wheat variety

- 4 ounces lean roast beef

- ½ cup arugula

- ¼ cup sliced cucumber

- 2 tablespoon Parmesan, grated

- 1 teaspoon balsamic vinegar

- 1 teaspoon olive oil

- black pepper, freshly ground

- dried oregano

Preparation:

- Get the pita bread. Pile it up with the roast beef, arugula, cucumber, and Parmesan.

- In a separate bowl, mix the olive oil and vinegar. Season it with pepper and oregano.

- Drizzle the dressing over the pita filling. Fold and cut into wedges.

Cranberry-Quinoa Salad

Ingredients (makes 4 servings):

- ¼ cup cranberries, dried

- 1 cup of quinoa, uncooked

- 2 cups of mixed greens (e.g. arugula, spinach)

- 2 pieces of scallions, chopped finely

- 1/8 cup of pine nuts

- ¼ cup of cashews

- 2 teaspoon miso paste

- ½ cup of water

- ¼ teaspoon of agave nectar

- 3 tablespoon lemon juice, freshly squeezed

- 1 tablespoon of lemon zest

- 2 cloves of garlic, minced

- ¼ teaspoon red pepper, crushed

- Salt and pepper, to taste

Preparation:

- Cook quinoa following package instructions.

- Combine the dressing ingredients in a blender, cashews, pine nuts, miso, nectar, water, lemon juice and zest, garlic, red pepper, season to taste with salt and pepper. Process until the consistency is good for salad dressing.

- Combine the quinoa, cranberries, mixed greens and scallions. Toss with the prepared dressing. Serve.

White Beans with Kiwi-Coconut Sauce

Ingredients:

- 1 medium-sized red onion, roughly chopped

- 1 tablespoon green curry paste

- 1 can (about 14 oz) of light coconut milk

- 11 pieces of kiwi fruits, peeled, chopped (makes about 4 cups)

- 1 can (8 oz) pineapple chunks, drained then chopped

- 1 can (15.5 oz) of cannellini beans, rinsed

- 6 tablespoon sunflower seeds

- 2 tablespoon chopped cilantro

- 3 tablespoon sliced shallots

Preparation:

- Lightly coat a skillet with oil and sauté onions until soft.

- Add curry paste, 1 1/3 cup of kiwi and coconut milk.

- Bring the mixture to a simmer. Cover the pot.

- Cook for 5 minutes, until the fruit is soft.

- Remove from heat and puree in a blender.

- Bring back the coconut mixture to the pot and simmer.

- Put all the remaining ingredients in a bowl. Mix thoroughly. Pour the kiwi-coconut sauce and serve.

Berry Power Smoothie

Ingredients (makes 4 servings):

- 2 cups of mixed berries

- 1 cup of Greek yogurt

- 1 piece banana, sliced

Preparation:

- Place everything in a blender and blend until smooth.

- Serve.

Orange vinaigrette

Ingredients (makes 4 servings):

- ¼ cup of freshly squeezed orange juice

- 2 tablespoon of balsamic vinegar

- 1 tablespoon of Dijon mustard

- 1 tablespoon raw honey

Preparation:

- Combine all the ingredients in a jar with a tight-fitting lid.

- Cover the jar and shake well until everything is well combined.

- Store in the refrigerator. It can last up to 1 week.

- Shake before serving.

- Use as dressing over salad greens.

Orange Rice

Ingredients (makes 4 servings):

- 1 ½ cups fresh orange juice

- 1 tablespoon butter

- 1 teaspoon orange zest, grated

- 1 ½ cups rice

- 1 can (11-ounce) mandarin orange (segments), drained

Preparation:

- Place a medium-sized saucepan over stove on medium-high heat.

- Place the butter, orange zest and juice. Bring the mixture to a boil.

- Stir in the rice.

- Cover and cook until the rice is done.

- Remove from the heat and rest for 5 minutes.

- Fluff the rice then mix the mandarin orange segments in.

- Serve warm.

Curried Pear and Butternut Squash Soup

Ingredients (makes 8 servings):

- 1 medium-sized butternut squash

- 2 pieces pears, firm and ripe, diced

- 2 tablespoons butter, unsalted

- 2 cloves of garlic, minced

- 1 medium onion, diced

- 1 tablespoon of curry powder

- 2 teaspoons of fresh ginger root, minced

- 1 teaspoon salt

- 4 cups chicken broth, low sodium variety

- ½ cup of half-and-half

Preparation:

- Preheat the oven to 375°F.

- Cut the squash lengthwise and remove the seeds and membrane. Roast in the oven with the cut side down until very soft. Scoop out the pulp and set aside.

- In a soup pot, melt the butter. Sauté the garlic, onion, ginger, salt and curry powder.

- Pour the broth and bring to a boil.

- Add the pears and squash. Cook until very soft.

- Place the soup in a blender. Pulse until smooth.

- Pour the soup back to the pot. Add the half-and-half.

Roquefort Pear Salad

Ingredients (makes 6 servings):

- 1 head of leaf lettuce, sliced
- 5 ounces crumbled Roquefort cheese
- 3 pieces of pears, diced
- 1 avocado, flesh diced
- ¼ cup sugar
- ½ cup of pecans
- ½ cup green onions, sliced thinly
- 1/3 cup of olive oil
- 3 tablespoon of red wine vinegar
- 1 clove of garlic, chopped
- 1 ½ teaspoon mustard
- ½ teaspoon of salt
- Black pepper, to taste

Preparation:

- Cook pecans with ¼ of sugar until the sugar caramelizes. Set aside on parchment paper.
- Create the dressing by mixing 1 ½ teaspoon sugar, garlic, mustard, oil, vinegar, pepper and salt.

- Layer pears, lettuce, avocado, cheese and green onion in a serving bowl. Pour the dressing over the salad. Top with the pecans.

Winter Fruit Salad in Poppy seed Lemon Dressing

Ingredients (makes 12 servings):

- ½ cup lemon juice

- ½ cup white sugar

- 1 teaspoon Dijon mustard

- 2 teaspoons onion, diced

- 2/3 cup vegetable oil

- ½ teaspoon salt

- 1 tablespoon poppy seeds

- 4 ounces shredded Swiss cheese

- 1 head romaine lettuce

- ¼ cup dried cranberries

- 1 cup cashews

- 1 pear, sliced

- 1 apple, diced

Preparation:

- Make the dressing by placing the lemon juice, sugar, salt, mustard and onion in a blender. Pulse until smooth. Slowly pour the oil while the motor is still on. Continue processing until well blended and smooth.

- Mix together lettuce (torn in pieces), cashews, apple, par,
cheese and cranberries in a serving bowl. Pour the dressing
and toss to coat.

Kiwi Smoothie

Ingredients (makes 4 servings):

- 3 pieces of kiwi, peeled then chopped

- 1 cup of blueberries

- 2 pieces of bananas

- 1 cup of plain Greek yogurt

Preparation:

- Mix everything in a blender. Process until smooth and well
blended.

Banana Boat

Ingredients (makes 2 servings):

- 2 bananas

- ¼ cup of miniature marshmallows

- ¼ cup chocolate chips, semisweet

Preparation:

- Make a slit along the length of the banana, careful not to
cut all the way through the bottom.

- Stuff marshmallows and chocolate into the slit.

- Wrap the banana in foil and cook over a barbecue fire, or bake until the chocolate melts.

- Serve warm.

Banana Smoothie

Ingredients (makes 2 servings):

- 1 fresh banana

- 1 ½ cups of almond milk

- ½ cup strawberries

- ½ cup mango chunks

- 1 cup spinach

- 2 tablespoons of Greek yogurt

- 1 tablespoon chia seeds

- 1 tablespoon of coconut oil

- 1 teaspoon bee pollen

Preparation:

- Mix everything in a blender until smooth and well combined.

Strawberry Kiwi Salad

Ingredients (makes 1 serving):

- 1 large kiwi fruit, peeled and sliced

- ½ cup strawberries, sliced

- ¼ cup plain Greek yogurt, non fat

- 1 teaspoon lime juice

- 2 teaspoon honey

- 1 tablespoon pistachios, chopped

- A sprig of mint

Preparation:

- Mix kiwi and strawberry slices in a bowl.

- In another bowl, mix yogurt, honey and lime juice. Spoon the yogurt mixture over the fruits.

- Top with pistachios and sprig of mint.

- Serve.

Chapter 9: **Superfoods For Increasing Brain Function**

Avocado Baked Eggs and Bacon on Toasts

Ingredients (makes 2 servings):

- 1 ripe medium (or large) avocado

- 2 bacon slices, cooked into a crisp then crumbled

- 2 pieces of small organic eggs

- 2 toast slices

- black pepper, freshly cracked

- sea salt, according to taste

- fresh chopped tomatoes, optional

- hot sauce, optional

Preparation:

- Preheat the oven to 425°F.

- In a separate medium-sized bowl, crack the eggs. Keep the yolks whole and intact. Set this aside.

- Take the avocado and cut it in half. Open it and remove the large seed. The resulting hole should be big enough to fit a small egg. If not, scoop out some of the flesh, a little at a time until the right size is achieved.

- Place the avocado in a baking dish. Make sure the avocado is stable and won't tilt over.

- Scoop one of the egg yolks with a spoon and carefully place it in the avocado hole. Add the egg whites until the hole is filled.

- Sprinkle salt and pepper over the egg according to preferred taste.

- Place the avocado in the oven and bake until the eggs are done. This may take about 15 minutes.

- Remove from the oven. Sprinkle the crumbled bacon on top of the eggs.

- Serve with toast and the optional tomatoes and hot sauce.

Peanut Butter Smoothie

Ingredients (makes 2 servings):

- 2 tablespoons of peanut butter

- 1 cup of plain yogurt

- ½ cup raspberries

- 1 banana

- 1 tablespoon cacao powder

Preparation:

- Mix everything in a blender. Process until well blended and smooth.

Blueberry-Lemon Syrup

Ingredients (makes 2-3 servings):

- ¾ cups of blueberries

- 2 teaspoons of maple syrup

- Juice of ½ of a lemon

Preparation:

- Mash the blueberries with a fork.

- Pour in the maple syrup and the lemon juice.

- Mix well.

- Serve over waffles or pancakes for a power breakfast.

Brown Rice Pilaf with Apricots and Mushrooms

Ingredients (makes 2 to 3 servings):

- 1 cup of brown rice, long-grain variety

- 2 cups of water or vegetable broth

- 2 teaspoons of extra-virgin olive oil

- 2 caps of Portobello mushrooms, chopped

- ¼ pound button mushrooms, sliced

- ½ of a small onion, roughly chopped

- Salt and black pepper, to taste

- ½ cup walnuts, toasted and roughly chopped

- ½ cup dried apricots, chopped

- ¼ cup fresh parsley and thyme, chopped

- ½ teaspoon of apple cider vinegar

Preparation:

- Sauté the mushrooms and onion in oil over medium high heat.

- Add the rice and water (or vegetable broth). Season with pepper and salt to taste.

- Reduce heat to simmer and cook for 45 minutes until all the liquid are absorbed by the rice.

- Remove the pot and let it sit for 10 minutes.

- Uncover the pot and fluff the rice.

- Transfer the rice to a large mixing bowl. Add the herbs, nuts, apricot and vinegar.

- Toss to combine well.

- Serve warm.

Pomegranate Juice

Ingredients (makes 1 serving):

- 2 to 3 pieces of pomegranate

- Seltzer or water

Preparation:

- Squeeze the juice from the fruit.

- Dilute with seltzer or spring water.

Brown Rice Salad

Ingredients (makes4 servings):

- 1 ½ cups of brown rice, uncooked

- 3 cups of water

- 2 tablespoon of balsamic vinegar

- 2/3 cup of fresh orange juice

- 2 tablespoons of vegetable oil

- 2 tablespoon orange zest

- 2 tablespoon raw honey

- ½ teaspoon salt

- 2 pieces large orange, cut into bite sizes

- 1 ½ cups packed spinach leaves

- 1/3 cup red onion, slivered

Preparation:

- Cook rice in water, about 45 to 60 minutes.

- Whisk together oil, orange juice, vinegar, orange zest, honey and salt. Pour this dressing over the cooked rice. Mix well, cover and chill.

- Stir in the spinach, onions and oranges just before serving.

Chocolate Blueberry Smoothie

Ingredients (makes 2 servings):

- 1 cup almond milk

- ½ cup yogurt

- ½ cup fresh or frozen blueberries

- ½ small avocado

- 3 Brazil nuts

- 1 tablespoon cacao powder

- 2 drops vanilla extract

- ¼ teaspoon cinnamon

Preparation:

- Blend together in a blender until smooth and creamy.

Coco-Choco Smoothie

Ingredients (makes 2 servings):

- ½ cup coconut milk

- ½ tablespoon coconut oil

- 1 cup almond milk, chocolate flavored or plain

- 2 medium-sized bananas

- 1 tablespoon chia seeds

- 1 tablespoon cacao powder

- ½ teaspoon vanilla powder or extract

Preparation:

- Mix in blender until smooth and well blended.

- Serve.

Cashew Smoothie

Ingredients (makes 2 servings):

- 1 cup coconut or almond milk

- 1/3 cup cashews

- 1 large banana

- A dash of cinnamon

- A dash of salt

Preparation:

- Mix everything in a blender until well combined.

Nut Bar with Dates and Almonds

Ingredients (makes 12 servings):

- 1 ¼ cups dates, pitted

- 1 cup almonds

- ¼ cup flaked coconut, sweetened

- ¾ cup crispy rice cereal

- ¾ cup apples, dried

- 1/8 teaspoon salt

- 1 tablespoon honey

- Cooking spray

Preparation:

- Place all ingredients except the cooking spray and cereals in a food processor.

- Process until everything is chopped finely. Add the cereals and pulse for a few cycles.

- Coat a glass or ceramic baking dish with cooking spray.

- Take the mixture and press into the baking dish.
- Cut into 12 even squares.

Sweet Potato with Apples and Cinnamon

Ingredients (makes 1 serving):

- 1 medium-sized sweet potato
- 2 tablespoons plain Greek yogurt, non fat
- 1 small apple, diced
- 1 teaspoon honey
- Dash of cinnamon

Preparation:

- Puncture the sweet potato with a fork then bake for 3-5 minutes.
- Slice the sweet potato in half.
- Top each half with yogurt, diced apple honey and cinnamon.
- Serve.

Salmon Cheese-and-Crackers

Ingredients (makes 4 servings):

- 1 small cheese wedge
- 4 whole grain crackers
- 1 tomato, sliced into 4
- Basil leaf

- Canned wild salmon, skinless and boneless

Preparation:

- Divide the cheese evenly and spread on the crackers.
- Top each cracker with a slice of tomato.
- Put a basil leaf on top of the cracker.
- Place about 1 ounce of salmon on the cracker.
- Serve.

Chapter 10: **Superfoods Recipes To Look Younger**

Spinach Salad

Ingredients (makes 4 servings):

- 5 cups of baby spinach

- 2 pieces of large eggs, hard-boiled, peeled and sliced into small wedges

- 2teaspoons lemon juice, freshly squeezed

- 2 tablespoons of extra virgin olive oil

- black pepper, freshly ground

- ½ teaspoon of kosher or sea salt

Preparation:

- Combine olive oil and lemon juice. Season to taste with pepper and salt.

- Place the spinach in a bowl and drizzle with the prepared dressing.

- Toss to coat the spinach evenly.

- Top with sliced eggs before serving.

Fettuccine with Wild Salmon and Strawberry

Ingredients (makes 2 servings):

- 1 9-ounce package refrigerated spinach or plain fettuccine

- 1 8-ounce salmon fillet, skinless and boneless

- 1/3 cup of raspberry vinegar

- 3 tablespoons of extra virgin olive oil

- 2 teaspoons of sugar

- ¼ teaspoon pepper, coarsely ground

- 1 clove of garlic, minced

- 1 cup strawberries, sliced in half

- ¼ cup green onions, sliced

Preparation:

- Whisk olive oil, raspberry vinegar and garlic in a small bowl. Season with salt and pepper, to taste. Reserve 1 tablespoon, set aside.

- Wash the fish and pat dry. Place on a broiler pan. Brush with the reserved 1 tablespoon of oil mixture. Broil the fish about 4 inches from the fire. Cook. The fish is done when it easily flakes using a fork.

- Cook the pasta according to package directions. Add salt to the water. Drain when al dente.

- Pour the oil mixture over the pasta. Toss gently to coat the pasta.

- Flake the salmon and add to the pasta. Toss gently.

- Top with sliced strawberries. Sprinkle with chopped green onions and serve warm.

Roasted Bell Peppers

Ingredients (makes 2 servings):

- 1 piece of medium-sized red bell pepper

- Olive oil

Preparation:

- Brush the red bell pepper.

- Roast until the skin starts to char.

- Remove all charred portions. Slice into strips and add to salads.

Apples with Yogurt Dip

Ingredients:

- 1 small apple, sliced

- ¼ cup plain Greek yogurt, nonfat

- 2 teaspoon honey

- ½ tablespoon peanut butter

Preparation:

- Make the dip by mixing the yogurt, honey and peanut butter.

- Dip the apple slices and enjoy.

Eggs on toast

Ingredients:

- 1 bread slice, 100% whole wheat variety

- 1 teaspoon olive oil

- Cooking spray

- 1 medium egg

- ½ cup baby spinach, fresh

- Salt, to taste

Preparation:

- Spread olive oil on the bread slice. Toast the bread until it turns golden brown.

- Spray a skillet with cooking spray and cook the egg. Sprinkle salt on the egg, if desired.

- Place the spinach on top of the toast.

- Put the eggs on top of the spinach.

- Serve warm.

Coconut oil and Strawberry Smoothie

Ingredients:

- 1 cup coconut milk

- 1 tablespoon of coconut oil

- 1 cup strawberries

- ½ tablespoon honey

- 1 large banana

Preparation:

- Blend everything in a blender until smooth.

- Serve.

Rosemary and Berry Sorbet

Ingredients:

- 1 tablespoon rosemary, fresh
- ½ cup wild blueberries
- ½ cup orange juice, freshly squeezed
- ½ cup green tea ice cubes (green tea frozen in ice cube trays)
- 2 tablespoons of chia seeds

Preparation:

- Mix everything in a blender.
- Serve immediately.

Tomato Penne

Ingredients:

- 8 ounces of penne pasta, cooked according to package directions
- 2 tbsp olive oil
- 2 cloves garlic, minced
- ¾ cup sun-dried tomatoes, chopped
- 1/3 cup walnuts, chopped
- ½ a block of firm tofu, pressed
- 1 teaspoon basil
- salt, to taste

Preparation:

- Mix the garlic, walnuts, basil, oil and tomatoes in a large bowl.

- Add the tofu and mash. Combine thoroughly.

- Add the sauce to the pasta. Toss until the penne is well and evenly coated.

- Serve warm or chilled.

Summer Greens on Bruschetta

Ingredients:

- 1 pound summer greens, washed and dried

- 3 tablespoons olive oil, extra-virgin

- ¼ cup toasted almonds

- 1 small onion, sliced thinly into rounds

- 1 garlic clove, minced

- 2 ounces of firm goat cheese, cut into 8 slices

- salt and pepper, to taste

- 2 teaspoons sherry vinegar

- 8 slices rustic bread, 1/2-inch thick and 4 inches across, toasted

Preparation:

- Place the almonds in a food processor and finely grind it. Set aside.

- Place a skillet over medium-high heat. Add 1 tablespoon of the olive oil.

- Sauté the onion until soft.

- Add the summer leafy greens.

- Season with salt and pepper.

- Cook the greens until soft and liquids have evaporated.

- Cool the greens then toss with vinegar.

- In another bowl, combine garlic and the ground almonds. Add the remaining olive oil (2 tablespoon). Season to taste with salt and pepper.

- On each bread slice (bruschetta), spread about 1 teaspoon of the almond mixture. Place a cheese slice on top. Lastly, top with the summer greens.

Spicy Tomato Soup

Ingredients:

- 1 14-ounce can of diced tomatoes

- 3 cloves of garlic, minced

- 3 tablespoons of olive oil

- 1 carrot, peeled and sliced thinly

- 1 small red chili, fresh or dried pepper

- 1 ½ cups of plain soy milk

- 1 tablespoon lemon juice, freshly squeezed

- Coarse salt and ground pepper, to taste

- Parsley leaves, for garnish

Preparation:

- Strain the tomatoes. Reserve the juice.

- Place the tomatoes in a shallow baking pan. Drizzle with olive oil. broil until the tomatoes are lightly browned.

- Combine the tomatoes, chili, garlic, soy milk, carrots, lemon juice and reserved tomato juice in a food processor. Puree everything until smooth and well blended.

- Pour into a saucepan. Boil the soup over medium heat. Reduce the heat to a simmer.

- Cook for 5 minutes.

- Season to taste with salt and pepper.

- Before serving, garnish with parsley leaves.

Tomato-Paprika Salad Dressing

Ingredients:

- ¾ pound ripe tomatoes

- ½ teaspoon paprika, mild

- 3 tablespoons of red-wine vinegar

- 1 clove garlic, chopped roughly

- 1-2 teaspoons light-brown sugar

- ¼ cup olive oil, extra-virgin

- salt and pepper

Preparation:

- Boil the tomatoes for 30 seconds. Cut in quarters, then remove the skin and seeds.

- Place the tomatoes, garlic, sugar, vinegar and paprika in a food processor. Puree the mixture until smooth.

- Keep the motor on and pour the oil is a thin and steady stream.

- Season to taste with salt and pepper.

- Use on salads.

Pomegranate Mocktail

Ingredients:

- ½ slice of a medium orange, cut into wedges

- 1/3 cup of pomegranate syrup

- Sugar

- Ice cubes

- small pomegranates

Preparation:

- Take the orange wedges and rub them over the rim of martini glasses.

- Invert the rim and dip it in sugar.

- Combine the pomegranate syrup and ice cubes in a martini shaker.

- Shake and strain into the prepared glasses.

- Garnish with small, fresh pomegranates

Apple Mocktails

Ingredients:

- ½ slice of a medium orange, cut into wedges

- 1/3 cup of apple juice concentrate, frozen

- Sugar

- Ice cubes

- Apple wedges

Preparation:

- Prepare the martini glasses with oranges and sugar.

- Place the apple juice and ice cubes in the martini shaker.

- Shake and strain into the prepared martini glasses.

Spiced Walnuts

Ingredients:

- 2 cups walnut halves

- 2 teaspoons olive oil

- 1 tablespoon honey

- 2 tablespoons sugar

- 1 teaspoon coarse salt

- 1/2 teaspoon ground coriander

- 1 teaspoon ground cumin

- 1/8 teaspoon cayenne pepper

Preparation:

- Take a large skillet and heat the oil, honey and water. Add the walnuts. Toss gently to coat the nuts.

- Sprinkle cayenne, coriander, salt, sugar and cumin over the walnuts.

- Cook while tossing and stirring frequently until the walnuts are lightly browned and well coated with the spices.

- Cool the walnuts on a baking sheet.

Conclusion

Thank you again for purchasing the book *Superfoods: Ultimate Superfoods Health And Diet Detox Guide! - Increase Metabolism, Natural Beauty And Health With 50 Powerful Natural Remedies And Recipes For Anti-Aging, Fat Loss, And More!*!

I am extremely excited to pass this information along to you, and I am so happy that you now have read and can hopefully implement these strategies going forward.

I hope this book was able to help you understand what superfoods are, what they can do and how to include them in your meals.

The next step is to get started using this information and to hopefully live a healthier life!

Please don't be someone who just reads this information and doesn't apply it, the strategies in this book will only benefit you if you use them!

If you know of anyone else that could benefit from the information presented here please inform them of this book.

Finally, if you enjoyed this book and feel it has added value to your life in any way, please take the time to share your thoughts and post a review on Amazon. It'd be greatly appreciated!

Thank you and good luck!

Preview Of:

<u>Natural Remedies!</u>

Natural Herbal Remedies And Beyond For Your Health And Natural Beauty!

Introduction

I want to thank you and congratulate you for purchasing the book, "Natural Remedies! - Natural Herbal Remedies And Beyond For Your Health And Natural Beauty!"

This book contains insight to the amazing world of natural herbal remedies and how incredible they can be for your health!

This day and age many people automatically turn to the traditional medical field for all of their health and beauty problems looking for the answers. Unfortunately, many times these solutions can also come with their own problems. Now you have two problems to be treated! The first one you were looking to take care and a myriad of other side effects you must now also treat.

Over the years I have begun to realize that this is a very common and many people are looking for additional, more holistic ways of treating minor issues that won't have them second guessing later. This is my motivation for creating this book and hope you will find many solutions to everyday problems, and live a much healthier and happy life!

Thanks again for purchasing this book, I hope you enjoy it!

Chapter 1: Natural Herbal Remedies: An Introduction

I am so happy you have decided to go down this journey with me and I hope you find what you are looking for! I want to take a moment to explain why I have structured this book in the way it is. First this book is meant to provide you with as much information with as little clutter as possible, because at the end of the day what you want is solutions to your problems, not some fancy way of saying it! So please don't get hung up if you feel that sometimes the text is just giving you the facts and not a lot of fluff, that is the way it is designed - so you can get the most out of it! Now let's get started!!!

What's so great about using natural remedies, you ask? There are many great things about it, often overlooked by people who are quite used to taking medication that's been prescribed to them or ones that they are most familiar with. There's nothing wrong with that, of course, but one needs to be mindful of the different side-effects that these chemicals may bring about. Many people turn to the use of these natural remedies (otherwise known as home remedies or folk medicine) for many of their ailments because of the fact that these are made out of natural ingredients. Herbs, vegetables and fruits are just a few of the most common ingredients used in these remedies. The best bit, however, is that many of these things can be easily found in an average kitchen.

But will it work? Well, if you consider the fact that throughout history people have used and relied upon these natural medicines, then the answer would be a solid yes. This was before modern medicine was invented and the use of synthetic drugs was propagated. It works but as to what extent, well, that varies from one individual to the next. For simple cures, however, even some doctors recommend their use instead of depending on over the counter medicine. Even in the food that we consume on a daily basis, there are healing properties that can help combat certain types of illnesses. It would be to our benefit if we harnessed it and used to as supplements to the medications that we're taking. In fact, if it happens to be potent enough, you can use it by itself. Research and studies do prove that many of these natural remedies possess properties that work in the same manner as synthetic medication.

How do you get started with it then? Well, first off, you would require a certain knowledge of which ingredients you need for a particular ailment. That's where this book is going to come in handy. We'll get more into the specifics later.

Spices, herbs and even fresh food can be used effectively when it comes to treating most ailments that can range from minor pains to even infections. These days, people would rely on antibiotics for these things. Those can be quite expensive, let's be honest, and in some cases, they can also cause adverse side effects if misused. There's also the fact that these antibiotics also end up killing the good or beneficial flora and fauna in our bodies, thus making recovery time lengthier than usual. In worst case scenarios, they can backfire and actually damage our immune system. With natural home remedies, however, you can avoid all of that. Besides treating the infection itself, it also helps in strengthening our immune system which makes it more capable of defending itself from other ailments. We also recover better with it as it readily promotes mending and healing of various aches and pains, as well as burns and wounds.

Besides medicine, you can also make use of home remedies to make your own mouthwash and if you're really good, toothpaste. Some people go to the extent of creating medicinal soaps that allow them to avoid mass marketed ones that might contain ingredients that they're allergic to, don't support or extremely harsh for the skin.

It takes a bit more work to achieve these, but if you're really keen, a few hours out of your day should be enough. So, if you have certain skin issues and want to give natural soap a try, look to the later chapters for instructions on how you can make some. Besides hygiene products, you might also want to try creating remedies for indigestion and constipation, both common problems for modern man considering the diet we all have. This would be good if you need to regularly take something in order to be able to move your bowel easily.

What else can these home remedies be used for? There's also some that you can make in order to help yourself or a loved one recover from the flu in a quicker fashion. You may also make teas that would help relieve a cough or a sore throat. A throat spray (typically used for asthma) can also be made through the use of natural ingredients that, when compared to a store-bought one, would be far cheaper.

We've already touched on it but these remedies aren't just meant for internal use only. Besides the soaps and the mouthwash, you can also create your own natural cleanser that would treat skin conditions such as acne. An antiseptic spray made from natural ingredients can also be concocted and this would be great for eliminating dermatitis, as well as killing bacteria from scratches or cuts. It can also effectively heal blisters.

Needless to say, there is a lot that one can do when it comes to home remedies. All you really need is a simple guide, as well as a few free hours for research. The more familiar you are with the benefits of a particular ingredient, the better you will be at making and mixing remedies.

Thanks For Previewing My Exciting Book Entitled:

"Natural Remedies: Natural Herbal Remedies And Beyond For Your Health And Natural Beauty!"

To purchase this book, simply go to the Amazon Kindle store and simply search:

"NATURAL REMEDIES"

Then just scroll down until you see my book. You will know it is mine because you will see my name "Sarah Brooks" underneath the title.

Alternatively, you can visit my author page on Amazon to see this book and other work I have done. Thanks so much, and please don't forget your free bonuses

DON'T LEAVE YET! - CHECK OUT YOUR FREE BONUSES BELOW!

Free Bonus Offer: Get Free Access To The www.LuxyLifeNaturals.com VIP Newsletter!

Once you enter your email address you will immediately get free access to this awesome newsletter!

But wait, right now if you join now for free you will also get free access to the "Anti-Aging Made Easy" free EBook!

To claim both your FREE VIP NEWSLETTER MEMBERSHIP and your FREE BONUS Ebook on ANTI-AGING MADE EASY!

Just Go To:

www.LuxyLifeNaturals.com

www.ingramcontent.com/pod-product-compliance
Lightning Source LLC
Chambersburg PA
CBHW070808290526
45795CB00002B/665